Our Toxic World: A Survivor's Guide

Kathleen Barnes

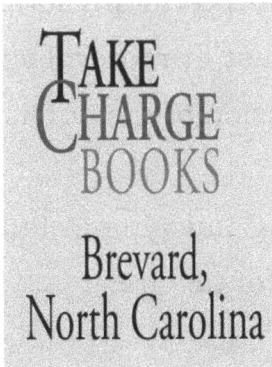

TAKE
CHARGE
BOOKS

Brevard,
North Carolina

The purpose of this book is to educate. It is not intended to serve as a replacement for professional medical advice. Any use of the information in this book is at the reader's discretion. This book is sold with the understanding that neither the publisher nor the author has any liability or responsibility for any injury caused or alleged to be caused directly or indirectly by the information contained in this book. While every effort has been made to ensure its accuracy, the book's contents should not be construed as medical advice. To obtain medical advice on your individual health needs, please consult a qualified health care practitioner.

Copyright © 2016 Take Charge Books, Brevard, NC.

Library of Congress Cataloging-in-Publication Data is on file with the Library of Congress.

ISBN: 978-0-9961589-3-0

Printed in the United States of America

10 9 8 7 6 5 4 3 2 1

Table of Contents

PART I
Toxins, Toxins Everywhere!

6

CHAPTER 1
We're Being Bombarded Every Day

We live in a toxic world. There is no way around it.

- The air we breathe is polluted. Outdoor air is polluted by industrial waste, dirty power plants, cars and trucks, industrial fumes and automotive exhausts. Automotive fumes and industrial waste have
- The water we drink is adulterated. Even when our municipalities claim is it "purified," it is riddled with toxic substances, including chlorine, fluoride and residues of prescription drugs.
- The food we eat has been altered to the point where our ancestors wouldn't even recognize it. Our food has been genetically modified, with carcinogenic additives and preservatives.
- Even the clothes on your back, the shampoos, toothpastes and skin creams you use, not to speak of sunscreens you use to prevent skin cancers, contain toxins and ingredients that cause cancer.

It sounds rather, grim, doesn't it?

After all, we all have to breathe, drink water, eat food and clothe ourselves.

It would be easy to feel overwhelmed and helpless.

But there are steps you can take to protect yourself and you family. In this book, I'm giving you simple, effective and reasonably priced ways to minimize or even eliminate your risk of toxic exposure in your daily life.

It would be easy to tell you that you need to move out of New York City, buy a farm in the middle of nowhere, get all your water from a well and grow all your food, but I realize this is not practical or even possible for many of us.

Resources are finite for most of us, so I'm going to give you the basic costs of healthier living and a list of priorities so you can make your choices and priorities.

Let's keep it real, my friends. First, by knowing the volume of pollutants that has infested our world, we can take the necessary steps to protect ourselves.

We do have choices in what we buy, what we eat and what we bring into our homes. To some extent, we can even choose our work environment and the school environments our children experience.

While none of us can single-handedly clean up the air or the water supply or the food production system, together we can have profound effects on the way things work.

I am a passionate believer in community and the collective voice of the people. At the risk of becoming overly political, I think it is fair to say that corporate interests most often get more attention from our government than do "We, the People." We can change that. It is time. It is our time.

Get involved. Call me crazy, but I attend almost all of our local government meetings. I go to the county commission meetings, if for no other reason than to let our elected representatives know that someone is interested, that their constituents are watching. I even attend county planning board meetings, which can be paralyzingly boring, with the occasional opportunity to make my voice heard.

A group of natural health advocates in our little city was able to stave off the City Council's attempt to re-introduce fluoride, a toxic chemical that disrupts hormone function, into the city water system.

By doing our homework, introducing carefully researched, irrefutable, scientifically validated information we were successful. This came in stark contract to local dentists who reflexively announced that cavities had increased in local children since fluoride was removed for the municipal water five years earlier. They didn't ask the most obvious questions: How much soda are these kids drinking? Where do they live? How many lives in houses on wells without fluoride and what is their cavity rate compared to kids who drink fluoridated city water?

To be frank, we beat the pants off the so-called medical professionals. The City Council voted 5-0 to keep fluoride out of our water. It was a sweet victory!

This is just one small example of how citizen participation can change the ways our elected representatives behave and profoundly influence our exposure to toxic chemicals.

This applies to local, state government and federal government. Take a few minutes and, if you don't already know your representatives, do a little research. Become your congressperson's pen pal. Ditto for your state legislators. Local elected officials are even easier to contact, since you're likely to see them in the supermarket or the local coffee shop as well as at regular meetings. Let them all know you care.

Elected officials must listen to their constituents if their voices are loud enough.

Find your senator here:

http://www.senate.gov/general/contact_information/senators_cfm.cfm

And your congressman/woman:

https://www.opencongress.org/people/zipcodelookup

And the president:

https://www.whitehouse.gov/contact

Just Google your state name and legislature for your state officials and search for your county and city websites to get contact into for your local officials.

Together, we will make a difference.

Part II
EARTH

Chapter 2
A Round Up of RoundUp's Lethal Effects

The cumulative evidence is indisputable: RoundUp is vastly harmful to human and animal health and to the environment. The evidence has become so overwhelming that I feel duty-bound to give you a list of the scientific studies that have been conducted that prove the harm caused by glyphosate, the major ingredient in RoundUp.

When you read it, you'll wonder along with me why the U.S. government allows this toxic chemical to be on the market, much less tolerates the vast agricultural use to which it has been put. Every single human being in North America has had deep exposure, whether or not we use RoundUp in our yards.

RoundUp probably won't kill you or your children immediately. You may have seen videos of Monsanto reps — I can only assume they are intellectually-challenged — who drink the stuff to demonstrate its "safety." I wonder what shape those guys and their kids (if they have any) are in now, 10 or 15 years down the road.

One such less-than-intelligent person who drank glyphosate immediately developed kidney failure and brain lesions and eventually went into a coma and died.

In any case, here's a summary of the research. I'm adding links to the scientific studies for those of you with deeply inquiring minds.

Underlying cause of obesity, diabetes, heart disease, cancer and more:

The truly frightening study published in 2013 in the journal *Entropy*, details the means by which glyphosate causes cell damage, interrupts the body's ability to detoxify environmental toxins and causes chronic inflammation, which, over time, results in a wide variety of our most dreaded chronic diseases.

Infertility and birth defects:

A group of scientists assembled a comprehensive review of existing data that shows European regulators have known since at least 2002 that glyphosate causes a number of birth malformations. Regulators misled the public about glyphosate's safety, and in Germany the Federal Office for Consumer Protection and Food Safety told the European Commission that there was no evidence to suggest that glyphosate causes birth defects.

This pivotal Canadian study suggests that increased prevalence of endometriosis coincides with the introduction of genetically modified foods and the glyphosate herbicides that go hand-in-hand with GMOs in "RoundUp ready crops."

A Columbian study showed a dramatically reduced pregnancy rates among women who lived in areas where glyphosate was aerially sprayed on crops versus those who lived in unsprayed areas.

And Brazilian researchers found that RoundUp exposure caused severe damage to sperm in lab rats and altered testosterone levels and reproductive development in prepubertal rats.

Cancer:

RoundUp exposure increases the risk of various types of cancer, including breast cancer, FIX LINK TO BREAST CANCER non-Hodgkins lymphoma and hairy cell leukemia.

Gluten intolerance and celiac disease: At least once study directly links the environmental toxicity of glyphosates with the worldwide epidemic of gluten intolerance and celiac disease.

Kidney and liver toxicity:

This damning French animal study showed not only vastly increased risks of kidney and liver damage among animals exposed to glyphosate, but also showed that the death rats in female rats tripled over non glyphosate-fed rats. This suggests that glyphosate is significantly more toxic to females than males.

Alzheimer's, Parkinson's and other neurodegenerative disorders:

Brazilian researchers, who have been at the forefront of the discovery of the toxicity of glyphosate, confirmed that the toxic herbicide causes brain cell disruption and can cause Alzheimer's disease, among other neurodegenerative disorders.

Chinese researchers found the mechanism by which glyphosate causes cell damage leading to Parkinson's disease.

This is just the tip of the iceberg, my friends. There is a great deal of scientific evidence that has convinced me without any doubt that glyphosate is a dire threat to our public health. The only beneficiary to the glyphosate glut is Monsanto. Follow the money and follow political contributions to legislators who will ensure Monsanto's protection.

Chapter 3
More Proof of Poison

RoundUp is everywhere. It's on your shoes, in your drinking water and in your food. This insidious poison is part of a greedy and misguided effort to completely control our food, engineered by Monsanto, to promote the sales of its GMO and RoundUp Ready seeds. The evidence is mounting. There's no longer any question that RoundUp is poison and that its use on food crops affects every single one of us.

Here's the latest:

"Probably carcinogenic"

The World Health Organization declared glyphosate, the active ingredient in RoundUp, is "probably carcinogenic to humans."

The world authority on cancer conducted a comprehensive review of the latest available research.

This puts glyphosate in the second highest category in terms of cancer risk. To put this in perspective, only about 100 substances worldwide are certified as carcinogenic to humans, the highest category. This means the WHO think there is a major cancer risk to humans from this weed killer that is everywhere, in your home yard and garden in your neighbor's garden and, worst of all, in commercial use.

Agriculture is the largest use of RoundUp worldwide, where it complements "RoundUp ready" GMO crops, primarily corn and soy that are used in almost all processed foods. It's also used in forestry, weed control in urban areas and along roadways.

Endocrine disruptor

Aussie lab research shows that glyphosate disrupts progesterone production in the amounts typically allowed in drinking water. Disruption of progesterone persisted after the glyphosate was removed.

Science has shown glyphosate is toxic and an endocrine disruptor in both men and women for more than five years. Summarizing their study, the authors of this French study said in the journal *Toxicology* in 2009, "A real cell impact of glyphosate-based herbicides residues in food, feed or in the environment has thus to be considered, and their classifications as carcinogens/mutagens/reprotoxics is discussed."

The Australian study is the first to show that RoundUp disrupts the production of progesterone.

Placental Cell Death

Glyphosate, this deadly poison also kills cells in the human placenta, the womb's guardian of unborn fetuses, not in unreasonable quantities, but at the levels allowed in U.S. drinking water.

If it kills placental cells, it stands to reason that it probably kills fetal cells, causing who knows what harm to the developing baby?

Breast milk!

If that's not enough, glyphosate has now been found in breast milk.

The study, conducted by the advocacy groups Moms Across America and Sustainable Pulse, showed glyphosate in breast milk at levels 760 to 1,600 times higher than the European Drinking Water Directive allows for individual pesticides, but lower than the 700 ug/l maximum level permitted by the EPA.

If you're breast feeding and you live in a city, it's likely your breast milk has toxic levels of glyphosate.

Drinking water and more

Had enough? Not yet? Try this one for size: glyphosate has also been found in the urine and drinking water of Americans at a level more than 10 times what is permissible by European standards.

The US geological Survey confirmed that herbicides, primarily glyphosate, have been found in 51 streams in nine Midwestern states.

Glyphosate gets into drinking water primarily through agricultural runoff into — you guessed it — streams and lakes.

There's more, but I'll leave you with this, for now:

At least six studies show that glyphosate causes birth defects, tumors and reproductive disorders in animals, even at dilutions far lower than those used in home gardening.

What can you do?

Don't buy or use RoundUp! Forward this article. Educate your friends, family and especially your neighbors. Write/call your congressman, senator, even the White House (see links in Chapter 1).

Make your voice heard: Glyphosate should be outlawed today!

Chapter 4
GMOs Increase Gluten Sensitivity

An important puzzle piece links GMOs (genetically modified organisms) found in a vast array of food products and gluten sensitivity. If you've dismissed friends who engage in the current "fad" of gluten intolerance, you may change your mind after reading this chapter.

A team of experts affiliated with the Institute for Responsible Technology says that GMOs and seeds inoculated with RoundUp™ herbicide and Bt-toxin insecticide trigger gluten-related disorders that affect 18 million Americans.

Gluten is found in wheat, rye and barley and can cause gluten sensitivity can cause symptoms ranging from gas and bloating to celiac disease, a serious autoimmune condition that can be life threatening.

A number of environmental links to gluten sensitivity have been proposed, including the higher gluten content of modern wheat strains (a 2013 review of data commissioned by the U.S. Department of Agriculture found no evidence to confirm this).

Other possible environmental factors in the dramatically increased incidence of gluten sensitivity include increased consumption of wheat and gluten products, the introduction of wheat to children at an early age, shorter breastfeeding duration, the current popularity of Cesarean birth that prevents the infant from being inoculated with beneficial bacteria in the mother's vaginal tract and general alterations in intestinal microflora in the population.

This is complex subject matter, so I'll try to make it as simple as possible. You're welcome to the full report at: http://responsibletechnology.org/glutenintroduction for yourself. There is an extensive list of references at the end of the article.

1. The U.S. Department of Agriculture, the Environmental Protection Agency and an array of research published in national and international medical journals links GM foods to five conditions that may either trigger or aggravate gluten-related disorders, including the serious autoimmune disorder, celiac disease:

- Intestinal permeability
- Imbalanced gut bacteria
- Immune activation and allergic response
- Impaired digestion
- Damage to the intestinal wall

2. There are nine GMO food crops currently being grown for commercial use: soy, corn, cotton (oil), canola (oil), sugar from sugar beets, zucchini, yellow squash, Hawaiian papaya and alfalfa. Wheat is not among them. Stay with me.

4. Most GMOs crops are engineered to tolerate a RoundUp, the weed killer also known as glyphosate. They contain high levels of this toxin at harvest. Research shows that glyphosate, even in very small doses, can significantly reduce the population of beneficial intestinal bacteria in humans and animals, and promote the overgrowth of harmful bacteria. This causes inflammation, leaky gut and immune reactions, all of which are linked to gluten-related disorders. Glyphosate also increases retinoic acid sensitivity, which has been shown to trigger gluten sensitivity.

5. Corn and cotton varieties are also engineered to produce an insecticide called the *Bacillus thuringiensis* or Bt-toxin. Bt toxin in GMO corn kills insects by punching holes in their digestive tracts and a 2012 study confirmed it punches holes in human digestive tracts, too. Bt-toxin has also been linked to overstimulation of the immune system and allergies.

Dr. Tom O'Bryan, internationally recognized expert on gluten sensitivity and celiac disease, says, "The introduction of GMOs is highly suspect as a candidate to explain the rapid rise in gluten-related disorders over the last 17 years."

Internist, Emily Linder MD, says, "Based on my clinical experience, when I remove genetically modified foods as part of the treatment for gluten sensitivity, recovery is faster and more complete. I believe that GMOs in our diet contribute to the rise in gluten sensitivity in the U.S. population."

How can we avoid GMOs? That's the million-dollar question since food manufacturers have been successful thus far in their well-financed campaign to prevent GMO labeling.

One answer: Eat entirely organic. If your budget can't accommodate that (mine can't!), avoid all foods on the GMO list, including the wide variety of processed foods that contain corn and soy. You'll have to be a careful label reader since so many related products are carefully disguised on ingredient lists. I'd love to hear from readers about your strategies for avoiding GMOs.

Chapter 5
Eating Bread? You're Eating RoundUp!

I've written loads of stuff about GMOs (genetically modified organisms) and the potential harm they can do us. Part of that harm is because GMO crops grown in the US are what they call RoundUp Ready.

That means that RoundUp, the broad-spectrum weed killer, can be sprayed on crops we want to keep and it will kill all the weeds around it without killing the food crop.

Now there's a new twist to the agricultural nightmare. Not only does RoundUp cause exponential growth of weeds that quickly become resistant, it's being sprayed on non-GMO crops as a desiccant to help dry them quickly.

You're probably way ahead of me and you've already guessed that it's being sprayed on wheat crops. While, thus far, wheat is not genetically modified, that doesn't prevent corporate greed from bringing wheat into the toxic brew.

RoundUp is also being routinely sprayed on other non-GMO crops, including barley, oats, canola, flax, peas, lentils, soybeans, dry beans and sugar cane.

That lovely green wheat blowing in the breezes will turn to "amber waves of grain" all by itself, but the agri-business powers that be have decided to speed up the process by spraying RoundUp on wheat crops, effectively killing and drying the plant quickly so the grain can be harvested.

Now we know that glyphosate, the active ingredient in RoundUp™ is an endocrine disruptor. It also has been linked to ADHD, Alzheimer's disease, autism, birth defects, several types of cancer, celiac disease and gluten intolerance, chronic kidney disease, colitis, depression diabetes, heart disease, hypothyroidism, leaky gut syndrome, liver disease, Lou Gehrig's Disease, multiple sclerosis, non-Hodgkin's lymphoma, Parkinson's disease, infertility, miscarriages and stillbirths, obesity and chronic respiratory diseases.

For more info and documentation on these, go to: http://ecowatch.com/2015/01/23/health-problems-linked-to-monsanto-roundup/

Here's the bad news. I don't want to hear it any more than you do: Any wheat product, except certified organic ones, contains RoundUp. That goes a long way toward explaining why glyphosate is present in nearly every human being in the Western world.

Chapter 6
Your Cotton T-shirt May Be Poisoning You

We all love our cozy cotton T-shirts, shirts, pants, underwear, towels and sheets. They feel comfy and safe.

The cotton industry fosters that illusion with its "fabric of our lives" campaign, pushing the notion that this "natural " fiber is healthy and creates happiness.

Nothing could be further from the truth.

Cotton is the most intensive pesticide-use crop in the world, accounting for approximately 25% of all insecticides used worldwide, although cotton is grown on only 3% of the world's farmland.

Five of the top nine pesticides used on cotton in the U.S (cyanide, dicofol, naled, propargite and triflurin) are known cancer-causing chemicals. All nine of the top pesticides used on cotton crops in the U.S. are classified by the EPA as Category I or II, the most dangerous categories of chemicals.

Cotton weevils are resistant to pesticides

The reason for the intensive pesticide use on cotton is that weevils and other cotton pests develop immunity to these chemicals very quickly, in about five or six years. It takes 8 to 10 years and approximately $100 million to develop new pesticides for use on cotton, so the new chemicals are ever more toxic and quickly become obsolete.

The cotton toxic waste is everywhere

In California, it has become illegal to feed the leaves, stems, and short fibers of cotton known as 'gin trash' to livestock, because of the concentrated levels of pesticide residue. Instead, this gin trash is used to make furniture, mattresses, tampons, swabs, and cotton balls. The average American woman will use 11,000 tampons or sanitary pads during her lifetime.

According to the Organic Consumers Association, about 80% of all the cottonseed and almost all the gin trash go right into feed for dairy cows and into our milk. The other 20% of the cottonseed is made into oil, meal and cake and winds up in many different junk foods.

Toxic substances are absorbed by skin

Cotton clothing places some of these pesticides right on your skin, which is the largest and most absorbent organ of your body. Not only is your skin in contact with that T-shirt, underwear or pants for most of the day, if you're sweating, the increased body heat can accelerate absorption of the pesticide residues in the fabric.

The problems with clothing production don't stop in the field. During the conversion of conventional cotton into clothing, numerous toxic chemicals are added at each stage— silicone waxes, harsh petroleum scours, softeners, heavy metals, flame and soil retardants, ammonia, and formaldehyde— to name just a few.

Other toxic clothing

Other common types of clothing aren't much better. Clothing made from synthetic fibers like acrylic, nylon and polyester is coated with formaldehyde finishes that continuously give off minute plastic vapors as the fabric is warmed against your skin, causing allergies and breathing problems from the airborne particles and unknown effects of formaldehyde in contact with large skin surfaces.

It's really no surprise that a recent study of the cord blood of 71% of newborn babies shows extensive exposure to toxic substances passed to the baby through the placenta, including some of those used in cotton production. Worse yet, the majority of these toxic substances are carcinogenic, 75% are toxic to the brain or nervous system and 72% cause birth defects or abnormal developments.

Healthy clothing

Clothing that is made from 100% organic cotton, silk, linen, hemp, or tencel (made from natural cellulose found in wood pulp) will be free of these toxic residues.

If all new clothing isn't in your budget, your old clothes may be OK or you can buy used clothing, which may outgas less since numerous washings may have removed some of the residues.

If none of these works for you, wash any new clothing several times before you wear it.

Chapter 7
Eeek! You're Putting What? Where??

While we're on the subject of what's touching your body, and especially your sensitive parts, consider feminine hygiene products, my sisters.

Skin is the body's biggest organ. We have 16 to 21 square feet of skin. And it's very absorbent. Consider the effectiveness of drugs like pain killers, nicotine withdrawal medications and even birth control delivered transdermally (through the skin). So your skin is quite literally drinking up anything that touches it.

Now think about the thin mucosal skin of your genitals, and even more so, your vagina. Whatever you put there ends up in your bloodstream and is distributed throughout your body.

Now think about what your skin may be absorbing from sanitary pads, panty liners, tampons, nursing pads for breastfeeding moms and, for those of who have passed into cronehood, incontinence products.

Health Guru Dr. Joseph Mercola calls feminine hygiene products a "ticking time bomb," estimating that the average American woman uses somewhere between 16,800 and 24,360 tampons in her lifetime.

What's in that pad or tampon?

It's important to note that manufacturers are not required to disclose the ingredients in their products. This undoubtedly includes pesticide-saturated cotton, plastic, dioxins (to bleach fibers white) synthetic fibers and petrochemicals. We're talking about bisphenol-A (remember that lovely little endocrine disruptor?), its' kissing cousin phthalate and any number of other odor neutralizers and leak stoppers.

Let's just take a brief look at dioxin alone. Fibers are naturally a buff color, but we've been conditioned to want our sanitary products to appear clean and white, so they are bleached with that Black Hat halogen, chlorine, which disrupts iodine absorption and, worse yet, creates dioxin, an endocrine disruptor that accumulates in fatty tissues and creates abnormal cell growth and suppresses the immune system. There is have no safe level of exposure to dioxin.

But that's not the end of it. We already know about the pesticides used to produce cotton. Well, my friends, most of the padding in these products is cotton. Add in the fact that almost all cotton produced in the US is genetically modified, and that also means it is saturated with RoundUp glyphosate, with all the negative health effects we've discussed at length.

There is also the risk of Toxic Shock Syndrome, a rapidly-multiplying bacterial infection that can be life threatening.

Inserting a couple of dozen toxin-laden tampons in your vagina every month may actually be worse than eating contaminated foods, since the skin so quickly and indiscriminately absorbs poisons into your body.

What to do?

Most of us aren't ready to go back to rag padding or anything so primitive. Many of us are also conscious of the environmental waste these products create.

Probably the easiest solution is a menstrual sponge. It's nothing more than a natural sea sponge. You can buy them at Walgreen's for $5 or even less at other online sources. Back in the day before my croning, I had three or four of them. You simply attach a piece of dental floss and it works exactly like a tampon, except you rinse them out and re-insert them. In between periods, boil them in water with a little vinegar to be sure there is no residual bacteria. Easy. Cheap. Effective!

There are also re-usable silicon menstrual cups like the Diva Cup made to be worn internally that trap the blood and are then washed out.

Organic cotton pads are available from companies like Natracare and Glad Rags and even organic unbleached tampons from Seventh Generation and Organyc offer a more traditional approach.

Chapter 8
They're Messing with Our Hormones

You may have heard the term "endocrine disruptor" applied to many substances that surround us every day, but maybe you didn't understand exactly what that means.

So here's your definition:

An endocrine disruptor is any substance that interferes with the endocrine (hormone) production system in mammals.

Yes, in simple terms, these things mess with our hormones. And when they mess with our hormones, endocrine disruptors can interfere with the immune system, cause cancer, birth defects, developmental disorders and infertility, not to speak of the accumulation of toxins in hormone-producing organs with unknown consequences.

The bad news is that endocrine disruptors are everywhere in our lives. The good news is that there is something we can do about it.

Here are some of the major ones:

Glyphosate: Numerous studies show the active ingredient in RoundUp herbicide causes substantial endocrine disruption, including lower progesterone levels, mammary tumors and severe organ damage, in levels permitted in drinking water, despite the US government's denial of its toxicity. It's also been linked to kidney disease, Alzheimer's disease, obesity, cancer and many more serous health problems. Some sources estimate as much as 80% of our food supply is contaminated with glyphosate, including many organic foods that are affected by drifting glyphosate sprays. Some scientists believe glyphosate may be the most toxic chemical ever approved for commercial use. It's difficult, almost impossible to avoid glyphosate. Avoid all wheat products, since even organic wheat has been contaminated, and wash your organic fruits and vegetables very carefully, with hydrogen peroxide, if possible.

Organophosphate pesticides: These chemicals developed for use in chemical warfare in World War II are still commonly used in pesticides today. They disrupt brain development, lower testosterone levels and cause thyroid hormone dysfunction. To avoid organophosphates, buy organic pest control products, don't let pest control companies into your home unless they are using completely organic products and can prove it and don't track outside residues into your home—leave your shoes at the door!

BPA (bisphenol-A): This chemical is used in most plastics and imitates estrogen in the human body. It's found in most canned foods and in thermal paper like that used in receipts, especially in plastics labeled polycarbonate.

Dioxin: Used in the production of paper and in many industrial processes, and has been documented to build up in the food chain and therefore in the human body, causing cancers, immune system and reproductive disorders. It's difficult to avoid dioxin, but the heaviest loads are in meats, fish, eggs and butter.

Atrazine: This herbicide is used on most corn crops and has contaminated much of the drinking water stored in open systems like reservoirs. It's been linked to breast tumors, prostate cancer and delayed puberty. Filter drinking water and buy organic produce to avoid atrazine.

Phthlates: Found in almost all soft plastics, including children's toys and shampoo and other personal care products, especially those with fragrances, phthalates are especially linked to changes in sperm count, less mobile sperm, birth defects in male babies, obesity, diabetes and thyroid dysfunction. Avoid plastic food containers and any personal care products that contain DEHP, DEP, DMP, BzBP and any artificial fragrances.

Perchlorate: This component in rocket fuel contaminates most of our fruits and vegetables and dairy products. Among its many health destroyers, it competes with essential iodine absorption and alters hormone production and metabolism and brain development in infants and children. If you don't have a well, filter all your water and install a reverse osmosis filter, which wastes an inordinate amount of water. Even organic foods can be contaminated; so adding iodine to your diet is essential to neutralize its effects.

Fire retardants: Most often found in children's sleepwear and polyurethane foam in furniture, fire retardants (polybrominated diphenyl ethers—PDBEs) are found in tissues and breast milk of people and animals worldwide. Several types of PDBEs have been phased out, but their residual effects are still found virtually everywhere. By imitating thyroid hormones, they disrupt the activity of real thyroid hormones resulting in variety of health problems, including lower IQs in children, reduced fertility and cancer.

Lead: We've all learned a lot more about the danger of lead due to the Flint, MI water crisis, especially because it causes brain damage. It also disrupts hormone activity, especially in the hormones that govern stress and cause high blood pressure, diabetes, anxiety and depression. Lead is still found in flaking lead-based paint in virtually all homes built before 1978, so it's important to keep painted surfaces smooth or even to remove old paint (an expensive and complicated procedure). Lead is also found in older plumbing pipes in homes and in municipal water systems, so test your water and install a whole house filter if you have elevated lead. Even that may not be enough, as residents of Flint, MI have found.

PFCs (perfluorinated chemicals): These chemicals found in non-stick cookware have been banned, but almost all of us have PFCs in our bodies and will show up in our bodies and those of our children for generations to come. PFCs never break down in the environment and causes decreased sperm quality, low birth weights in babies, kidney disease, thyroid disease and high cholesterol.

PART III
WATER

Chapter 9
Scary Stuff in Your Tap Water

Our drinking water is full of scary stuff, not the least of which is prescription drugs that make their way from human bodies though the sewage system, filtration and arrive back in our taps diluted, but more or less intact.

Yuck, you say? Yes, yuck.

You see, we're a nation of prescription drug junkies. It (almost) goes without saying that what goes in comes out, so those who pop pills in the morning and they come out during the day and are flushed right into our water system. Some of us even flush unneeded medications down the toilet, further contributing to the concentration of prescription drugs in the water supply.

Three important studies took a deep look at the problem of pharmaceuticals in municipal drinking water.

The first, in 2006, scientists at the Southern Nevada Water Authority decided to check out the theory that folks who drink municipal water are being exposed to pharmaceuticals in amounts that could cause health problems.

They looked at drinking water that services 328 million Americans and tested for 51 compounds in addition to the expected toxic chlorine and fluoride.

Here's what they found:

• Atenolol, a beta-blocker used to treat cardiovascular disease

• Atrazine, an organic herbicide banned in the European Union, but still used in the US, which has been implicated in the decline of fish stocks and in changes in animal behavior

• Carbamazepine, a mood-stabilizing drug used to treat bipolar disorder, amongst other things

• Estrone, an estrogen hormone secreted by the ovaries and blamed for causing gender-bending changes in fish

• Gemfibrozil, an anti-cholesterol drug

• Meprobamate, a tranquilizer widely used in psychiatric treatment

• Naproxen, a painkiller and anti-inflammatory linked to increases in asthma incidence

• Phenytoin, an anticonvulsant that has been used to treat epilepsy

• Sulfamethoxazole, an antibiotic used against the Streptococcus bacteria, which is responsible for tonsillitis and other diseases

• TCEP, a reducing agent used in molecular biology

• Trimethoprim, another antibiotic

A World Health Organization (WHO) study published in 2011 confirmed those finding and those concerns.

Then a 2014 Environmental Protection Agency (EPA) study looked at the drinking water of 50 of the country's largest waste treatment plants representing about 15% of the treated wastewater in the country. They found concentration of 56 active prescription drugs *at far higher concentrations than scientists had expected.*

The toxic soup included aspirin, acetaminophen, Viagra, statin drugs, codeine and other pain killers.

Worse yet, the analysis showed a high concentration of endocrine disrupting drugs, including birth control pills and other hormonal drugs, including estradriol, the drug that stops ovulation in most birth control pills and tamoxifen, the drug given as part of the long-term treatment for breast cancer.

Blood pressure medications were the highest concentrations in drinking water, the EPA found, followed by antibiotics.

The EPA researchers expressed concerns that antibiotic residues found in drinking water could contribute to antibiotics resistant bacterial strains, something that is already a major health problem.

Environmental experts note that hormone disruptors have profound effects on aquatic and plant life at extremely low levels, and no one knows yet at what level the drugs become toxic to humans or how they interact with other pharmaceuticals in water and in an individual's prescription regimen.

To add fuel to the fire, a subsequent study found concerning levels of methadone, narcotic used to lessen the symptoms of drug withdrawal and to treat chronic pain. A chemical reaction takes places when methadone interacts N-nitrosodimethylamine (NDMA), a chemical commonly used in water disinfection and becomes a potent cancer--causing compound.

Ay yi-yi! It might make you want to adopt the Charlie Chaplin water regimen: Never drink water because .... I'll leave the rest for now.

Now, I'd be remiss if I didn't say that the concentrations are extremely low and probably don't pose a risk for most healthy people. EPA scientists that a person who drinks two liters of municipal water a day might accumulate about one dose in an entire year, but they concede that the effects on infants, children, people with compromised immune systems or metabolic disease are unknown.

We also have no idea of the long-term effects of consuming all of this mish-mash at once. Knowing that drugs interact with each other all the time, it's not out of the scope of possibility that we are creating some really serious problems here.

What to do:

Sadly, if you are stuck drinking municipal water, you don't have a lot of choices. Even the most sophisticated filtration equipment is unlikely to be able to filter out all the pharmaceuticals.

A reverse osmosis water filter might help, but I can't find any solid evidence to confirm that. Bottled spring water is another option. Be sure the label says "spring water." Many bottled water products are nothing more than tap water.

That's another of many reasons why we live in the country and get our water from a deep well. If you can't move to the country, maybe you should consider making a move to the countryside a long=term life plan. In the meantime, maybe you have a friend who will let you fill water jugs from her well water.

Chapter 10
Fluoride in Water: Involuntary Medication

Well-informed communities knowledgeable about the toxic effects of water fluoridation are beginning to reject the outdated idea that mass medication will somehow prevent oral and dental problems.

Fluoridation is a practice of adding fluoride (a toxic agricultural waste product) to municipal water supplies. I consider it involuntary medication with a wide variety of harmful side effects. Unlike any other water treatment procedures, water fluoridation does not treat the water, but it absolutely affects the person consuming it.

The World Health Organization (WHO) acknowledges that there is little difference in the rates of tooth decay in children living in fluoridated and non-fluoridated communities. In fact, the U.S. is the only Western country that permits fluoridation of water supplies. All of Europe, Japan and Korea prohibit water fluoridation.

In addition, the Centers for Disease Control and Prevention confirms that topically applied fluoride, as in fluoridated toothpaste, may have a positive effect in preventing cavities, but ingested fluoride, as in drinking water, has little, if any, positive effect and plenty of negative ones.

Why reject fluoride?

Fluoride is toxic, pure and simple. The Centers for Disease Control and Prevention confirms that one-third of American children have dental fluorosis (discolored teeth) caused by excess fluoride consumption. Excess fluoride consumption has also been linked to bone fractures, behavioral problems, hypothyroidism, bone cancer and reduced IQ in children.

The fluoride myth

Since the early 1950s, fluoride has been promoted by government and dentists alike as a solution to cavities, tooth decay and other dental problems in children.

Major dental problems being acquired by our children are rooted in high consumption of sugar and poor dietary habits. I am talking about the buckets of sugar (or more accurately deadly high fructose corn syrup)-laden Coke with which many of our children (and adults) wash down their meals. Parents and health educators are remiss in teaching good nutrition proper dental hygiene.

We would all be better served by a government that promotes proper dental hygiene and dietary habits instead of spending taxpayer money adding toxic chemicals to our water supply.

If you're still drinking the Fluoride Myth Kool-Aid (pun intended), by all means buy fluoridated toothpaste. It may help and it probably won't hurt much unless you swallow it (please note the warning label). For the rest of us, we'll cherish our clean pure water, thank you very much.

Chapter 11
White Hat and Black Hat Halogens

Note: This chapter is compliments of Dr. Robert Thompson, author of
What Doctors Fail to Tell Your About Iodine and Your Thyroid (To Your Health Books).

Now is a great time to take a deeper look at the dangerous dance of halogens in our bodies.

Iodine is a halogen, like the other chemical elements, bromine, fluorine and chlorine and their derivatives bromide, fluoride and chloride.

Iodine is the only one that has health benefits for humans. It's the good guy wearing the white hat, while its destructive brothers are the bad guys in the black hats, hell-bent on blocking your body's ability to absorb and utilize the iodine that is essential to life:

- Chlorine is now almost universally used to purify municipal water supplies instead of iodine. Even if you don't drink municipal water, if you shower or bathe in it, you are exposed to its toxic effects. Perchlorate, a highly toxic chlorine derivative used for rocket fuel among other things, has become pervasive in the water supply.
- Fluoride is now found in almost all toothpastes and municipal drinking water supplies. Some unenlightened dentists still insist on fluoride treatments to prevent tooth decay, despite the fact that there is no scientific evidence that the application of this toxic waste product has any positive effects. Fluoride has been confirmed to interfere with thyroid function and has been associated with some types of cancer.

- Bromine or bromide, also known to cause cancer, replaced iodine in commercial baked goods and almost all flours more than three decades ago. You'll also find potassium bromide in soft drinks, plastics, cans and jars, many personal-care products, sprayed on fruits and vegetables to inhibit mold, especially berries, in electronics and it has also been added to some vaccinations and asthma inhaler medications to replace mercury as a preservative. There are few or no labeling requirements. It's impossible to avoid breathing bromine fumes in any house, car, school or office building, so we are all continuously exposed to this cancer-causing chemical.

Other iodine robbers

Recently, we've also learned that soy-containing foods in some circumstances may block your body's ability to use iodine, and, with the increasing epidemic of gluten sensitivity, there are signs that gluten may also block iodine absorption.

This all adds up to a conspiracy on the part of the Black Hat halogens and their partners in crime, soy and gluten, to rob your body of its ability to use iodine to complete millions of vital metabolic functions every day.

The Black Hat halogens compete with White Hat iodine for access to your cellular function. Each cell has receptors, which function just like locks. All halogens have the keys to these locks—and the Black Hats do everything they can to prevent White Hat iodine from opening the locks.

How to avoid Black Hat halogens

Here are a few ways to avoid bringing any more Black Hat halogens into your home and your body:

1. Avoid all products made with brominated flours. Even products made with organic flours may contain bromine, since it is considered a natural substance. I know of only one brand, King Arthur Flour, which is not contaminated with bromine. Look for the words "non brominated" on the label to be sure. Bromine is also found in many soft drinks, wine and beer.
2. If you have a municipal water system, invest in a whole house water-filtration system to prevent absorption of halogens through your skin when you shower.
3. Don't use fluoridated toothpaste.
4. Avoid soy and gluten as much as possible.
5. Don't eat or drink food that is stored in plastic containers.
6. Avoid soft drinks.
7. Look for chemical-free personal-care products.
8. Ventilate your home and your workspace well. Open windows whenever weather permits.

We owe a great deal to Dr. Guy Abraham, the UCLA professor who pioneered iodine research through the Iodine Project for this information about toxic halogens and much more.

Iodine supplements

Nearly everyone needs some level of iodine supplementation and most of us need a lot of it to get to optimal iodine levels (90% excretion on a 24-hour loading test).

The good news is that iodine, the White Hat halogen, can fight back and overcome the Black Hat chlorine, fluorine and bromine molecules, crowd them off the cell receptors and be back in the game with access to your cells, if you get enough. It takes a lot of iodine to counteract and reverse the effects of bromine.

It is virtually impossible to get enough iodine from food and table salt.

The answer is to find the best possible supplement, one that offers iodine in three important forms, each with its own benefits:

- Potassium iodide for thyroid health
- Sodium iodide for thyroid, prostate, pancreatic, brain and immune system health
- Molecular iodine from kelp for breast, ovarian, prostate and reproductive system health

Note: Some people are "allergic" to iodine. This almost always means they are allergic to the organic form of iodine, such as the Betadine that is used in hospitals. It is nearly impossible for a human to get too much dietary iodine. Excess iodine is just excreted through the urine when it is not needed. There is no known toxicity for iodine except untreated cases of hyperthyroidism. For those who experience symptoms of intolerance (such as diarrhea or stomach upset), start with small doses and gradually build up to the optimal dose.

PART IV
SURVIVOR'S TOOLKIT

Chapter 12
The myth of organic food

Organic food is good for you and good for the planet. Most of my readers would agree on that point.

In the U.S., organic foods are subject to federal regulations that govern how the foods can be grown, raised and processed.

Definition of organic foods

In general, organic foods and livestock must be grown without the use of non-organic pesticides, insecticides and herbicides. Livestock must be raised without the routine use of so-called prophylactic antibiotics (an oxymoron if there ever was one!) and fed a generally healthy diet.

Processed organic foods (another oxymoron, in my opinion) must be free of artificial additives and preservatives and they must not result from genetically modified ingredients or be subjected to food irradiation or chemical ripening.

What a wonderful toxic soup!

Here are other differences between conventional farming and organic farming:

Conventional farmers:

Apply chemical fertilizers to promote plant growth.
Spray insecticides to reduce pests and disease.
Use chemical herbicides (mainly RoundUp and toxic glyphosates) to manage weeds.
Give animals antibiotics, growth hormones and medications to prevent disease and spur growth.

Organic farmers:

Apply natural fertilizers, such as manure or compost, to feed soil and plants.
Use beneficial insects and birds, mating disruption or traps to reduce pests and disease.
Rotate crops, till, hand weed or mulch to manage weeds.
Give animals organic feed and allow them access to the outdoors. Use preventive measures — such as rotational grazing, a balanced diet and clean housing — to help minimize disease.

Organic food is now big business

Until the 1990s, organic food growers were largely Mom and Pop farms and their produce was sold in local farmers markets. Not only were these farms sustainably operated, the food traveled a short distance from farm to market to table and was therefore environmentally sound and highly nutritious.

Now organic food and beverages count as the fastest growing segment of the U.S. food industry with upwards of $39 billion in annual sales in 2014—two and one half times the reported sales in 2008.

As a result, the organic food movement has become big business. With that comes the baggage of agribusiness, including shaky standards full of loopholes, including the import of so-called "organic" ingredients from other countries with few, if any, organic certification standards.

Organic food is higher in nutrients

Organic food is good for you. Research shows organic food contains 50% more nutrients, minerals and vitamins than produce that has been intensively farmed. It's questionable whether that is still true in view of the mega farming practices that include soil-depleting intensive single crop production and dairy operations where cows rarely if ever, see the light of day.

Organic food may not be organic at all

Buyer beware: Organic food isn't all it's cracked up to be.

You can pretty much trust foods that contain only one ingredient. Fruits, vegetables, eggs, dairy products and meat that are labeled 100% organic have fulfilled the ever-more-lax USDA certification standards and are marked with a small "USDA Organic" seal.

However, foods that contain more than one ingredient, like cereals or bread are much more complex. Read your labels carefully:

• A food is 100% organic only if it contains label that specifically says so.
• If a food carries a "USDA Organic" label, it means that 95% of the ingredients are organically produced. The other 5% is anybody's guess.
• Worst of all, if the label says, "Made with Organic Ingredients," that means the product must contain at least 70% organic ingredients. In other words, 30% can be non-organic and contain artificial preservatives, additives and other harmful substances.

Organics are more expensive

Organic food is generally more expensive than conventionally produced food, largely because of the labor-intensive farming methods necessary to produce organics.

However, many supermarket chains now carry private label "generic" organic foods at more affordable prices and there are supermarket chains like Aldi's and Trader Joe's that have made deep commitments to sustainable and organic products.

Consider the pesticide load

If your budget won't permit going entirely organic, consider the chart below to help you decide which foods are worth the expenditure:

Here's the list of the **DIRTY 50**, from worst to best non-organic produce:

Strawberries
Apples
Nectarines
Peaches
Celery
Grapes
Cherries
Spinach
Tomatoes
Sweet bell peppers
Cherry tomatoes
Cucumbers
Snap peas—imported
Blueberries—domestic
Potatoes
Hot peppers
Lettuce
Kale/collard greens
Blueberries—imported
Green beans

Plums
Pears
Raspberries
Carrots
Winter squash
Tangerines
Summer squash
Snap peas-domestic
Green onions
Bananas
Oranges
Watermelon
Broccoli
Sweet potatoes
Mushrooms
Cauliflower
Cantaloupe
Grapefruit
Honeydew melon
Eggplant
Kiwi
Papaya
Mango
Asparagus
Onion
Sweet peas frozen
Cabbage
Pineapple
Sweet corn (if non-GMO)
Avocado

--from the Environmental Working Group

I have to add a personal note here: I know coffee is technically a vegetable. Certainly it is a staple of life for many of us. However, coffee is not included on the above list.

Coffee is one of the most pesticide intensive crops in the world. If you're a coffee lover like I am, consider lowering your toxic load by buying organic coffee, better yet shade grown and fair traded to add to the eco-friendly perks. (Pun intended!)

My bottom-line advice

1. Shop the perimeter of your supermarket. Base your diet almost exclusively on fresh fruits, vegetable, dairy products and meats. You might make a brief detour down the aisles for nuts, organic grains and oils. Frozen vegetables and fruits are sometimes cheaper and have lower pesticide loads.

2. Buy organic as much as your budget will allow and use the "dirty 50" list to help you make your choices when you can buy organic.

Chapter 13
Docs call for GMO labeling

Mainstream medicine is entering the fray on GMO labeling, on the side of those of us who think we ought to have a right to know what is in our food.

In an article published recently in the usually stodgy *New England Journal of Medicine,* doctors from Harvard, Mt. Sinai Medical Center and the University of Wisconsin say that the pesticides applied to GMO crops (RoundUp ready) pose a risk of cancer. They urge the government to abandon its resistance to GMO labeling (heavily funded by Monsanto, producer of GMO seeds and RoundUp) in the interest of consumers' right to know what is in our food.

". . . the argument that there is nothing new about genetic rearrangement misses the point that GM crops are now the agricultural products most heavily treated with herbicides and that two of these herbicides may pose risks of cancer," wrote Mt. Sinai's Dr. Philip Landrigan and University of Wisconsin's Dr. Charles Benbrook.

The authors further urge the EPA to deny the approval of a new herbicide combo, designed to address increasing pesticide resistance in agricultural crops, because of recent studies that indicate the pesticide, Enlist Duo™, adversely affects the health of infants and children from glyphosate (RoundUp) a "probable human carcinogen" and 2,4-D, a "possible human carcinogen.

"These classifications were based on comprehensive assessments of the toxicologic and epidemiologic literature that linked both herbicides to dose-related increases in malignant tumors at multiple anatomical sites in animals and linked glyphosate to an increased incidence of non-Hodgkin's lymphoma in humans," the authors wrote.

They added that glyphosate resistant weeds are now found on 100 million acres of agricultural land in 36 states, so Monsanto wants to add 2, 4-D, an ingredient of Agent Orange defoliant used in the Vietnam War and linked to a wide array of health problems, including generational genetic problems passed from Americans who fought in Vietnam in the '60s and '70s.

More than 90% of corn and soybeans produced in the United States is genetically modified.

The only way to be certain that the food you are buying is not genetically modified is to buy USDA certified 100% organic products.

Chapter 14
The Right Seeds

If you're anything like me, you spend some of those cold, blustery winter evenings leafing through a stack of garden catalogs, dreaming of the gardens to come.

While we have a lot of space to garden, I know my gardening dreams become a bit larger than my energy levels. By mid-summer and I am sending psychic barbs at those enticing seed catalogs, as I battle the July weeds that have sprouted higher than my head.

Nevertheless, this year's quest has been for non-GMO seeds.

A few years back, GMO giant Monsanto began gobbling up seed companies like there is no tomorrow. It now controls approximately 40% of the global seed market. If Monsanto gets its way, there are questions whether there will be a tomorrow or a world for our children and grandchildren.

It is to everyone's benefit to keep Monsanto out of our gardens as well as off our tables.

Monsanto grabbed 20% of the global seed market in 2005 when it bought out Seminis, the largest developer, grower and marketer of fruit and vegetables in the world.

Seminis, under Monsanto's auspices, supplies the genetics for 55% of the lettuce on U.S. supermarket shelves, 75% of the tomatoes and 85% of the peppers, with strong holdings in beans, cucumbers, squash, melons, broccoli, cabbage, spinach and peas.

If this sounds like a dark conspiracy to control the world's food supply, I won't argue with you.

So this year's quest for my own garden has been for non-GMO seeds and those sold by companies not controlled by or supplied by Monsanto. It's a lot harder than you might think.

While heirloom and certified organic seeds might be free of GMOs, they may be sold by companies related to Monsanto in some way, therefore you can't be sure.

For example, Seminis' non-GMO seeds are carried by many popular garden catalogs, including Park Seed, Burpee, Territorial Seeds, and Johnny's Selected Seeds. I've noticed this year that Burpee's seeds contain a "non-GMO" label, but buying from Burpee still means you are indirectly giving money to Monsanto.

It gets even more diabolical: So Monsanto is buying up seed companies whose products are the result of generations of research and labor by traditional agricultural methods.

Then they can slip a "Round-Up Ready" or other proprietary gene into it and call it their "own", and sell it with patent restrictions. This means that Monsanto can eventually control the entire global seed market and — oh horrors!– control the entire world food supply. Forget about politics, he who controls food controls the world.

Sorry. Maybe I got a little carried away there. Or not.

Down to the heart of the matter:

- Buy from this list of companies that Monsanto HASN'T bought and are not affiliated with or do business with Seminis. NOTE: This list is a postcard. Other links seem to have mysteriously disappeared from the web. The Occupy Monsanto list has disappeared and the website (occupy-monsanto.com) seems to be abandoned for the past year. Hmmm.

- Avoid certain heirloom varieties because Monsanto now apparently owns the names (not necessarily the seeds, just the names).This article http://cleanfoodearth.blogspot.com/2012/03/keep-this-seed-names-list-monsanto.html) lists the seed varieties to avoid.
- Ask seed companies if they have taken the Safe Seed Pledge. Here's a list of companies that have done so: http://www.councilforresponsiblegenetics.org/ViewPage.aspx?pageId=261
- Avoid seeds of plants at big box stores that carry Seminis or Monsanto names on their labels. This includes some of the most popular tomato varieties like 'Celebrity,' 'Early Girl' and 'Better Boy,' as well as other common home garden varieties, like 'Cheddar' cauliflower, 'Marketmore 76' cucumbers and my favorite "Blue Lake 7' green beans.

Chapter 15
Toxic Personal Care Products

Toxic exposure is inevitable unless we can learn to live without breathing, eating or interacting with any substances around us. If you've figured out how to do any of those, please let me know your secret!

Several studies now show us that fetuses are exposed to toxins in the womb. We like to think of our newborns as pure and perfect, but studies from the U.S. Environmental Working Group published ten years ago showed 287 environmental toxins, industrial chemicals, pesticides and cancer-causing substances in the cord blood of newborns. They also now have a cool new tool that lets you look up your favorite products: http://www.ewg.org/skindeep/

Today, I'd just like to take a look at our morning routines and the numbers of toxic exposures we all get in the course of simply getting ready to leave the house for the day.

The Basics

What you put *on* your body is just as important as what you put *in* your body.

- Your skin is the largest organ of your body. It is porous, so what you put on the outside of your skin is quickly absorbed into your entire system. Think of your skin more as a sponge than as a barrier.
- Clothing made from natural and organic fibers prevents your skin and lungs from being in contact with toxic substances and vapors.

- Basic personal care products ranging from soap to toothpaste to shampoo are loaded with potentially dangerous chemicals.
- Cosmetics are particularly easily absorbed because they are typically put on our most fragile skin and, in the case of facial makeup, they remain on our bodies for hours at a time and they contain a wide array of toxic substances.

Basic personal care items most of us use every day can pose a serious danger to you. Worst of all, many of these toxic substances are not listed on labels, or they can actually be added to products labeled as "natural."

Here's a short list of the most dangerous:

1. **Pthalates:** Those petrochemicals used to make rigid plastics soft and pliable, are also commonly added to cosmetics. Pthalates are linked to elevated rates of endocrine disruption, increasing the risk of breast cancer and other hormonally-related cancers in both men and women. Perfumes, nail polishes, lotions, hair sprays and many other body care products contain phthalates also labeled DBP and DEHP. DBP is used extensively in body care products and DEHP is present in many household products, which we'll address in the next chapter.
2. **Parabens:** Another type of hormone disruptor commonly used in shampoos, conditioners, moisturizers. They are xenoestrogens—false estrogens—that interrupt the fertility cycle and can lead to early puberty in children.
3. **Sodium laureth sulfate:** You'll find it in shampoo, body wash, toothpaste, household cleaning products. Originally made as a pesticide, when combined with other common chemicals, it can form cancer-causing nitrosamines.

4. **DEA (diethanolamine) MEA (monoethanolomine), TEA (triethanolamine):** Commonly found in shampoos, soaps, bubble baths and facial cleansers. These are all hormone disruptors, with a strong link to liver and kidney cancer.
5. **Propylene glycol:** This is antifreeze—found everywhere in shampoos, cosmetics, conditioners, toothpaste, stick deodorants–and ice cream. It's linked to kidney and liver disease.
6. **Petrolatum (minerals oil and paraffin):** This base of cream, baby rash ointments and many other personal care products coats the skin like plastic, causing toxins to accumulate, disrupting hormonal activity, increasing the risk of cancers and accelerating skin aging.
7. **Formaldehyde:** Found in body lotions, shampoos and conditioners, body washing style gels, sunscreens, makeup and nail polish, formaldehyde is a known human carcinogen that is toxic to the immune system and respiratory tract.

This list is far from a complete list, but it gives you the idea of the level of toxicity we encounter in the most basic products most of us use daily.

What to do

Toothpaste: Most toothpastes have fluoride, an industrial waste product that disrupts thyroid activity and can cause a rare form of bone cancer. Many toothpastes also include petrochemicals, artificial colors and mineral oil that can cause a wide range of debilitating symptoms, including extreme fatigue, muscle pain, respiratory problems and possibly cancer.

The fix: Baking soda or fluoride-free natural toothpastes are a better choice.

Shampoos: Shampoos are commonly made with formaldehyde as a preservative, often labeled quaternium-15, a carcinogen that is also an irritant to skin, eyes and respiratory passages, even in small amounts. Although the government requires some products to carry a warning label, shampoo is not included.

Many shampoos (and body washes and bubble baths) contain chemicals that look like an alphabet soup called BNPD, TEA and DEA that can combine at random to form carcinogenic nitrosamines. Since nitrosamines are easily absorbed through the skin and your pores are open because you're using hot water, it's best to avoid products containing them.

Dandruff shampoos usually contain selenium sulfide, which can cause vital organs to degenerate if swallowed. Resorcinol, another easily absorbed ingredient in dandruff shampoos, can cause skin and eye irritation, drowsiness, unconsciousness and convulsions.

The fix: There are dozens of brands of non-toxic shampoos. My favorite is Dr. Bronner's, a 100% organic product that is gentle on skin and hair. You can also find organic shampoos, although many are only 80 or 90% organic, leaving you to wonder what's in that other 10 or 20%. Baking soda is the best topical remedy for dandruff.

Soap: Many soaps contain petroleum-derived synthetic fragrances, artificial colors, and mineral oil that may cause skin rashes and other allergic reactions.

The fix: Look for vegetable oil-based soaps or castile without artificial fragrances.

Deodorant: Ordinary deodorants can be a source of harmful chemicals. Virtually all antiperspirants have aluminum chlorhydrate, the active ingredient that prevents wetness that can cause infections in the hair follicles and skin irritations that may be severe enough to require medical attention. It is possible that the aluminum in deodorants may also contribute to the buildup of aluminum in the body, since aluminum from other sources has been linked to brain disorders and Alzheimer's disease. Aerosol sprays containing aluminum chlorhydrate can also be inhaled, potentially worsening the problem.

The fix: There are lots of natural deodorants. Just walk through the natural body care aisle at your local health food store and you will see a wealth of choices. Plain baking soda works well, even for people with strong body odor. The deodorant crystal-stone available in natural food stores are made from crystallized minerals, including alum, not aluminum. They're very effective and though they are a bit pricey, one stone will last for years.

Chapter 16
The Right Personal Care Products

On my recent wondrous trip to Peru's Amazon River basin, we stayed in a retreat center far from any city. There was electricity only for a handful of hours a day from a generator and no waste disposal system. Because of the delicate ecology of this most precious part of our planet, we were asked to use only organic and biodegradable personal care products.

This wasn't much of a problem for me, since I have been an avid label reader and researcher into the toxic chemicals that surround us every day, often in places we don't notice. Our morning bathroom routine is probably among the most toxic. I read somewhere that most of us have been exposed to 78 toxic and possibly cancer-causing chemicals by the time we finish showering and brushing our teeth each morning.

I don't have any way of verifying those numbers, but I do know that the shampoos, shower gels, toothpaste, deodorant, toilet paper and even the water we use, are all incredibly toxic.

If you want further information on toxic personal care products, I recommend the Environmental Working Group's site (http:www.ewg.org/skindeep)

I've done almost everything necessary to minimize the toxins in my personal care products. I long ago ditched deodorants that contain aluminum, shampoos, soaps and body washes with parabens, BPA and a wide variety of carcinogens, toothpaste with endocrine-disrupting fluoride. I recently banished endocrine disrupting nail polishes.

But my trip to Peru presented a unique problem: Not only was I deeply committed to respecting the sacred soil of the Amazon region, I would be traveling for nearly three weeks and I need something completely biodegradable and non toxic that would serve multiple purposes for washing hair, body, teeth and clothes.

My quest took me to Google, of course, where I re-discovered an old friend: Dr. Bronner's castile soap. Any castile soap will probably do, this is just one that brings back fond memories with its iconic cluttered label replete with a wealth of wise advice.

My grandmother used it. I used it for a while in my younger years and then moved on to other products. The Dr. Bronner's website (www.drbronner.com) calls them "magic soaps," for a good reason.

By definition, castile soap is made without the animal fats used in most soaps. It's basically olive oil, water and sodium hydroxide. Some formulations add essential oils, including peppermint, which makes it a bit more palatable as a toothpaste substitute.

Dr. Bronner's website boasts that its organic fair trade product can be used for "washing your face, body, hands and hair, for bathing, shaving, brushing your teeth, rinsing fruit, aromatherapy, washing dishes by hand, doing laundry, mopping floors, all-purpose cleaning, washing windows, scrubbing toilets, washing dogs, controlling dust mites, and killing ants and aphids" and more. I can personally attest to many of these claims.

This pretty much filled the bill for our trip to Peru. One medium-sized bottle to take care of everything I needed (no need for dog shampoo or toilet cleaning on this trip, but certainly when we got home).

It did everything I needed and didn't dry out my somewhat cantankerous skin and hair, even without conditioner. I did try it out beforehand to be sure I wouldn't have a haystack on my head for those obligatory vacation selfies. It washed my clothes, cleaned my teeth and worked as shaving cream.

And it's cheap. I was able to buy a half-gallon bottle for just over $30, which I subdivided into an 8-ounce container for the trip. I'm guessing it will take another year to use up the rest of that bottle, maybe somewhat less after my laundry experiment with it. It's also very concentrated, so a few drops do the job.

We're happily home from a wonderful trip, but Dr. Bronner's is back in my cabinet and it will replace many other products I no longer need.

Chapter 17
More Safe, Natural and Economical Beauty Products

It's not just what you put *in* your body, but what you put *on* it that can have a profound effect on your health.

It sometimes shocks me to see people who wouldn't dream of eating processed foods slathering on chemical-laden moisturizers or sunscreens. What you put on your body is just as important as what you put in it. It's just that many of us don't realize that skin is the largest human organ and that is it very permeable, meaning is easily absorbs anything you put on it.

Have you read the labels in your bathroom lately? What's in your shampoo? Your conditioner? Your moisturizer? Makeup? Soap? Toothpaste? If you aren't aware of the chemical names for cancer-causing chemicals and endocrine disruptors that are rife in personal care products, you'll probably be shocked.

I've developed a couple of simple solutions to the dilemma of what to put on my skin:

1. Don't use it on your skin if you wouldn't eat it.
2. Don't buy it if you can't pronounce all the ingredients easily.

You don't have to spend hundreds of dollars or knock yourself out to find safe, natural personal care products. Most health foods stores now have personal care and cosmetic lines that don't have these dangerous chemicals.

But it can be even easier than that. Here are a few of my favorites:

Organic Coconut Oil: Coconut oil has a multitude of uses. This is a wonderful moisturizer. It's a little oily, so I have to wait about half an hour after I put it on before the shine disappears. It's also a great cuticle softener and nail strengthener, easily breaks down calluses (rub a little on your feet and then put on socks) and even is a good treatment for dry scalp and hair. A 64-ounce container set me back just $13 and it will last easily for two years.

Witch hazel: Grandma's do-everything astringent, witch hazel tightens skin, dries oil skin and treats acne, cools down sunburn and eases the itch of contact dermatitis, hemorrhoids and bug bites or stings. I wouldn't be without it! And it's also ridiculously cheap. A 16-ounce bottle sells for $7 or less at your local pharmacy and will last easily for a year or more.

Baking soda (sodium bicarbonate): Baking soda makes a great toothpaste and breath odor neutralizer. It's also a skin exfoliant and is excellent for removing excessive hair product from over-processed hair. Many people substitute baking soda for deodorant with mixed success. Ask your friends if it's working! It cleans ground-in dirt from hands and nails and softens skin. It also eases itching due to bug bites or other skin irritations plus a host of household cleaning uses too numerous to mention here. And it's so cheap it's barely worth mentioning the cost: about 89 cents a pound that will last for months.

Chapter 18
Give up glitzy nails? Oh, no!

I'm a girly girl and I nearly always have nail polish on my toenails. Not on my fingernails, mind you, since they get wrecked in no time in the garden and in the barn. But I just love the sight of pretty toes.

But now I'm re-thinking that little personal indulgence based on some new research from Duke University and the Environmental Working Group that says we absorb endocrine disrupting chemicals from most nail polishes.

The study in *Environment International*, found that all 26 women in the study had a metabolite of triphenyl phosphate, or TPHP, in their bodies just 10 to 14 hours after painting their nails. Their levels of diphenyl phosphate or DPHP, which forms when the body metabolizes TPHP, had increased by nearly sevenfold.

The study included 10 commonly used nail polishes and the toxic chemical was found in 8.

Endocrine disruption means that the chemical interferes with normal hormone function and can cause reproductive and developmental irregularities.

TDHP (sometimes called TPP) is a chemical also used in fire retardants in foam furniture and plastics manufacturing.

Worst of all, there are no labeling requirements for TPHP or DPHP, so it's very difficult to know if you are messing yourself up by having pretty toes or fingers.

It's also very disturbing that these products are being marketed as safe, when they clearly are not (like fragrances, cosmetics and personal care products, but that's a story for another day). Even worse, my young granddaughters love to paint their nails and their mom's and mine.

The goods news is that there is an excellent resource to determine if your favorite nail polish is toxic and to find one that's not. The Environmental Working Group has an extensive database of cosmetics, including nail polishes. Click here to find out what's good and what's not. (www.ewg.org/skindeep/browse/nail+polish) Warning—sometimes EWG forces you to give up your e-mail address or even solicits a donation in order to see the info and sometimes not. I find that extremely annoying, but there is a workaround–just Google "safe nail polish" and an open link will come up.

Here's a synopsis of the bad guys:

- Sally Hansen (ouch—my fave because it is so tough)
- OPI
- Wet N Wild
- Revlon
- Beauty Without Cruelty

Among the safer nail polishes are:

- Aquarella (Expensive! $18 a bottle!)
- Piggy Paint (much more reasonable–about $8 a bottle)
- Poofy Supernaturals (seems to be available only throught its website, https://www.poofyorganics.com/search.aspx?searchterms=nail+polish)

Remember, toxicity also includes base coat, which is probably the most important since it is indirect contact with your bare nail, so be sure you're getting a safe base coat as well.

Find more info on the study at:
http://www.ewg.org/research/nailed/nail-polish-chemical-doubles-furniture-fire-retardant

Chapter 19
Get Your House Green and Clean

What is it about the early parts of the year when I want to clean out clutter, sweep away old papers and cobwebs and get the house good and clean?

Whatever it is, any time is a great time to have a clean and green house.

What's good for you is good for the Earth. And what's good for the earth is good for you.

I often have conversations with people who want to keep toxic chemicals out of their homes and to save money at the same time.

Voila! I have an answer for you!

You can clean almost anything in your home with seven ingredients. You probably already have most of them in your kitchen.

- Vinegar
- Baking soda
- Borax
- Lemon juice
- Olive oil
- Vegetable-based liquid soap
- Washing soda

Many people seem to think that cleaning naturally is expensive and inconvenient. Nothing could be farther from the truth. It's cheap. It's easy and it's effective. AND you're not exposing yourself to a toxic soup that includes allergens, carcinogens, neurotoxins, hepatotoxins, central nervous system depressants that can cause everything from liver failure to life-threatening allergic reactions to cancer to death.

We are all exposed to toxins every day. We can't avoid them. Research tells us that even newborn babies already have nearly 300 toxic substances in their bodies, passed on from their mothers. Over our lifetimes, that toxic load builds and builds until, one day, the balance may be tipped into toxic overload.

So if you can reduce your toxic load as much as possible, you can avoid that toxic overload, and postpone or even overcome existing toxic overload.

Back from my toxin rant: Natural cleaning products work. They are safe, easy and cheap. What's not to love?

What could be simpler than combining ½ teaspoon of vegetable-based oil, 3 tablespoons of vinegar and 2 cups of water in a spray bottle to make your windows sparkling clean for a nickel a bottle? Add a few drops of lemon essential for long-lasting shine, a great scent and to help energize the window washer!

How about scrubbing sinks, tubs and showers with a gentle paste of baking soda and borax? It works just as well as commercial cleaners with no toxic fumes and again, it costs mere pennies.

Pour a cup of borax in your toilet and leave it overnight. That's all it takes to wipe out my least favorite household task. Add a few drops of tea tree, lavender or white thyme essential oil for disinfection.

If your oven is an embarrassment like mine can be, try this:

Sprinkle water in the bottom of your oven, then cover the yuck with baking soda. Sprinkle some more water on top and let it sit overnight. In all but the worst cases, you'll be able to simply wipe it clean the next morning. If there is still stubborn baked-on grease, add a little washing soda to the mixture to cut the grease. Rinse well.

The best book I've read on non-toxic cleaning is Annie Berthold-Bond's *Clean and Green.* Annie's website is http://www.anniebbond.com.

A final thought about being clean and green: All of these recipes are nontoxic and they don't require any power tools. If you have a truly untenable stain or grease splotch, you might consider buying a Scunci steam cleaner. It uses nothing but water. In fact, you'll damage it if you try to add any cleaners to it and the superheated water will clean just about anything for a few pennies worth of electricity.

Chapter 20
Take Off Your Shoes!

Do you take your shoes off at the door? It's not an Eastern or hippie-dippy thing to do. It makes good, common sense.

Just think about where your feet are during the day:

You've walked on city sidewalks that have been salted and sprayed and perhaps slathered with dog poop.

You've crossed city streets that are saturated in hydrocarbons from cars and trucks, droplets of oil and other bodily fluids of petro-fueled vehicles and who knows what else.

You've probably shuffled across synthetic office carpets saturated with petrochemicals and perhaps even bearing the detritus of toxic chemicals used in the manufacture of pressed board furniture, including formaldehyde.

After a long day, you thankfully return home. Perhaps you took a little walk around your yard, admiring the newly planted petunias and pulling a stray weed along the way. Did you know that most yards are saturated with toxic chemicals, not the least of which is the endocrine disruptor RoundUp? You don't use RoundUp, you say? Does your neighbor? You don't know and you can't control your neighbor's activities anyway and your neighbor's RoundUp can become a part of your yard with just a little gust of wind.

Maybe you're really lucky like I am, and you can walk through your neighboring properties or a local park, enjoying the woods and the joys of nature. What toxic chemicals have been used there? Our neighbors are very vigilant about keeping toxic chemicals off our mountains, well, all except one, anyway, who raises cattle and uses a wide variety of toxic agri-chemicals that inevitably run down onto everyone's property. What's more, the power company came in and ransacked hundreds of trees they thought would threaten power lines, sealing the deal by spraying industrial strength RoundUp on everything to prevent re-growth.

Here's my point: Despite our best efforts, we all walk on toxic chemicals every single day. Why bring them into your house where they are re-circulated through heating and cooling systems?

It's easy to put a shelf just inside your front door and convince family, friends and visitors to stash their shoes. If you want to be especially kind, you can even provide slippers or flip-flops for those who prefer not to go barefoot. It'll go a long way toward reducing your toxic exposure.

Chapter 21
Take Heart

I'm the first to admit this book is far from comprehensive. This subject is so vast and so fluid that we learn of new dangers and new threats every single day.

I know there are gaps here. We could talk more about the neonicotinoid pesticides that are threatening our bee population, unwillingness on the part of Congress to force food manufacturers to label GMO products, the scourge of disposable diapers for infants and adults, contaminated prescriptions drugs and vaccines that have cast effects on our health and so much more. I promise I will address these and more in my newsletter and blog, www.kathleenbarnes.com/newsletter.

Baby steps

Yes, I understand that all of this information may seem overwhelming. But you know how to eat an elephant? One bite at a time.

Take baby steps. They will have a great effect on your life and your health. You may not be able to incorporate every suggestion I make, so do what you can. Add something extra from time to time.

Please take heart! If you've read this book closely, you know that there are many things you can do to protect yourself and your family from the dangers of Our Toxic World.

Knowledge is power. You now have some powerful tools to lessen the impact of toxins in your food, your home and your life. You also have the power, along with me and thousands of my readers, to forge the change we all need to protect ourselves and our planet.

You don't have to break the bank or rob one

Many people think non-toxic living is expensive. That depends on your savviness as a shopper. You can pay $15 for a bottle of laundry detergent or $3 for a box of washing soap that is just as effective and not harmful to you or the environment. Yes, I have a friend who makes bucketsful of non-toxic, effective laundry detergents for a couple of dollars.

Yes, organic food is often more expensive, much more expensive than non-organic food. Again, as a savvy shopper, you can find bargains.

I live in Brevard, NC, a very small town (population 6,000, 40 miles from the nearest city). Yes, we can get some organic products locally, but we can't get everything we need. I make time to travel to Asheville, the closest big city, once a month or so where I can take advantage of bargains at Aldi, Trader Joe's and Earth Fare. Yes, it takes a few hours of my time, but it's worth it to me. I usually combine the rip with lunch with friends or something fun.

I also order some things online--especially supplements and staples like Himalayan sea salt. I grow most of our produce in the summer and preserve what I can for winter.

I consider the time and money investment in our health as an important expenditure. I'd rather spend my money on good food than on medicines, surgeries and declining health. Wouldn't you? Let's get on the clean living bandwagon together.

REFERENCES AND RESOURCES

Chapter 2: A Round Up of RoundUp's Lethal Effects

Potrebic O, Jovic Sotsic J et al. Acute glyphosate-surfactant poisoning with neurological sequels and fatal outcome. *Vojnosanit Pregl.* (article in Serbian) 2009 Sep;66(9)758-62.

Samsel A, Seneff S. Glyphosate's Suppression of Cytochrome P450 Enzymes and Amino Acid Biosynthesis by the Gut Microbiome: Pathways to Modern Diseases. *Entropy* 2013, *15*(4), 1416-1463;

Aris A, Paris K. Hypothetical link between endometriosis and xenobiotics-associated genetically modified food. *Gynecol Obstet Fertil.* (article in French) 2010 Dec;38(12):747-53.

Sanin LH, Carrasquilla G et al. Regional differences in time to pregnancy among fertile women from five Colombian regions with different use of glyphosate. *J Toxicol Environ Health A.* 2009;72(15-16):949-60.

Dallegrave E, Mantese FD et al. Pre- and postnatal toxicity of the commercial glyphosate formulation in Wistar rats. *Arch Toxicol.* 2007 Sep;81(9):665-73.

Romano RM, Romano MA et al. Prepubertal exposure to commercial formulation of the herbicide glyphosate alters testosterone levels and testicular morphology. *Arch Toxicol.* 2010 Apr;84(4):309-17.

Thongprakaisang S, Thiantanawat A et al. Glyphosate induces human breast cancer cells growth via estrogen receptors. *Food Chem Toxicol.* 2013 Sep;59:129-36.

Eriksson M, Hardell L et al. Pesticide exposure as risk factor for non-Hodgkin lymphoma including histopathological subgroup analysis. *Int J Cancer.* 2008 Oct 1;123(7):1657-63.

Hardell L L. Eriksson M et al. Exposure to pesticides as risk factor for non-Hodgkin's lymphoma and hairy cell leukemia: pooled analysis of two Swedish case-control studies. *Leuk Lymphoma.* 2002 May;43(5):1043-9.

Seralina GE, Clair E et al. Long term toxicity of a Roundup herbicide and a Roundup-tolerant genetically modified maize. *Food Chem Toxicol.* 2012 Nov;50(11):4221-31.

Samsel A, Seneff S. Glyphosate, pathways to modern diseases III: Manganese, neurological diseases, and associated pathologies. *Surg Neurol Int.* 2015 Mar 24;6:45.

Ya-xing G, Xiao-ning F et al. Glyphosate induced cell death through apoptotic and autophagic mechanisms. *Neurotoxicology and Teratology.* 34;3, 2012 May–June: 344–349.

Chapter 3: More Proof of Poison

Cressey D. Widely Used Herbicide Linked to Cancer, Scientific American, March 25, 2015

Gasnier C, Dumont C et al. Glyphosate formulations induce apoptosis and necrosis in human umbilical, embryonic, and placental cells. *Toxicology.* 2009 Aug 21;262(3):184-91.

Gasnier C, Dumont C. et al. Glyphosate-based herbicides are toxic and endocrine disruptors in human cell lines. *Toxicology.* 2009 Aug 21;262(3):184-91.

Bus JS. Analysis of Moms Across America report suggesting bioaccumulation of glyphosate in U.S. mother's breast milk: Implausibility based on inconsistency with available body of glyphosate animal toxicokinetic, human biomonitoring, and physico-chemical data. *Regul Toxicol Pharmacol.* 2015 Dec;73(3):758-64

Glyphosate in drinking water: http://toxics.usgs.gov/highlights/glyphosate02.html

Ho MW. Glyphosate herbicide could cause birth defects. *Science in Society* 43, 36, 2009.

Chapter 4: GMOs Increase Gluten Sensitivity

Sapone A, Bai JC, Ciacci C et al. Spectrum of gluten-related disorders: consensus on new nomenclature and classification. *BMC Med.* 2012;10 13.

Kasarda DD. Can an increase in celiac disease be attributed to an increase in the gluten content of wheat as a consequence of wheat breeding? *J Agric Food Chem.* 2013;61 (6):1155-1159.

Yuan Y, Xu W et al. Effects of genetically modified T2A-1 rice on the GI health of rats after 90-day supplement. *Sci Rep.* 2013;3:1962.

Chapter 5: Eating Bread? You're eating RoundUp!

Report from government of Alberta, Canada:

http://www1.agric.gov.ab.ca/$department/deptdocs.ns
f/all/faq7206?opendocument

http://ecowatch.com/2015/01/23/health-problems-
linked-to-monsanto-roundup/

http://www.realfoodhouston.com/wp-
files/2014/11/14/is-glyphosate-monsantos-roundup-
used-on-wheat/

Chapter 6: Your Cotton T-shirt May Be Poisoning You

http://www.ecochoices.com/1/cotton_statistics.html

http://www.organicconsumers.org/clothes/224subsidie
s.cfm

http://www.ewg.org/reports/bodyburden2/execsumm.
php

Corssan AN, Kennedy IR. Calculation of pesticide
degradation in decaying cotton gin trash. _Bull Environ
Contam Toxicol._ 2008 Oct;81(4):355-9. 9414-9.

Chapter 6: Eek! You're Putting What? Where?

Archer JC, Mabry-Smith R et al. Dioxin and furan levels
found in tampons. _J Womens Health (Larchmt)._ 2005
May;14(4):311-5.

Chapter 8: They're Messing With Our Hormones
Myers JP, Antoniou MN et al. Concerns over use of
glyphosate-based herbicides and risks associated with

exposures: a consensus statement. *Environ Health.* 2016 Feb 17;15(1):19.

Schang G, Robaire B et al. Organophosphate Flame Retardants Act as Endocrine-Disrupting Chemicals in MA-10 Mouse Tumor Leydig Cells. *Toxicol Sci.* 2016 Apr;150(2):499-509.

Cruz G, Foster W et al. Long-term effects of early-life exposure to environmental oestrogens on ovarian function: role of epigenetics. *J Neuroendocrinol.* 2014 Sep;26(9):613-24.

Annamalai J, Namasivayam V. Endocrine disrupting chemicals in the atmosphere: Their effects on humans and wildlife. *Environ Int.* 2015 Mar;76:78-97.

Chapter 9: Scary Stuff in Your Tap Water

WHO report on pharmaceuticals in drinking water
http://www.who.int/water_sanitation_health/emerging/info_sheet_pharmaceuticals/en/

https://www.epa.gov/water-research/concentrations-prioritized-pharmaceuticals-effluents-50-large-wastewater-treatment

http://www.newscientist.com/article/dn16397-top-11-compounds-in-us-drinking-water.html

Chapter 10: Fluoride in Water: Involuntary Medication

Fluoride in drinking water WHO report:
http://www.who.int/water_sanitation_health/publications/fluoride_drinking_water/en/

CDC report on dental fluorosis:
http://www.cdc.gov/nchs/products/databriefs/db53.htm

Chapter 11: White Hat, Black Hat Halogens

Find a good biochemistry book. It's all there. I promise.

Chapter 12: The Myth of Organic Food

USDA Organic standards:
https://www.ams.usda.gov/rules-regulations/organic

EWG Dirty 50:
https://www.ewg.org/foodnews/list.php

Chapter 13: Docs Call for GMO Labeling

http://www.nejm.org/doi/full/10.1056/NEJMp1505660

Landrigan P, Benbrook C. GMOs, Herbicides, and Public Health. N Engl J Med 2015; 373:693-695.

Chapter 14: The Right Seeds

Occupy Monsanto:
Occupy-monsanto.com

Monsanto owned:
http://cleanfoodearth.blogspot.com/2012/03/keep-this-seed-names-list-monsanto.html

Chapter 15: Toxic Personal Care Products

EWG Personal Care Products database:
http://www.ewg.org/skindeep/

About the Author

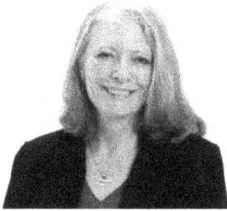

Kathleen Barnes has been an ardent advocate of natural health since the days when yoga was weird and taking vitamin C was considered "way out there." How times have changed!

Her career as a journalist and writer has spanned more than four decades, including years as an international correspondent for ABC and CNN during historic transitions in the Philippines and South Africa.

In recent years, she has turned her writing to natural health and sustainable living, writing and editing more than 20 books, many of them through her publishing company, take Charge Books.

She has written extensively for national and international publications, including more than six years as the weekly natural health columnist for *Woman's World* magazine and currently as a contributing writer to *Natural Awakenings* magazine.

Kathleen lives in the Blue Ridge Mountains of western North Carolina with her husband, Joe, and an ever-changing extended family of horses, dogs, cats and the occasional pond frog.

Other Books by Kathleen Barnes

Food Is Medicine: 101 Prescriptions from the Garden (Take Charge Books, 2015)

The Calcium Lie 2: What Your Doctor Still Doesn't Know with Dr. Robert Thompson (Take Charge Books, 2013)

10 Best Ways to Manage Stress (Take Charge Books, 2013)

Eight Weeks to Vibrant Health: A Take Charge Plan for Women with Dr. Hyla Cass. (Take Charge Books, 2008 second edition, first edition McGraw-Hill).
The Calcium Lie: What Your Doctor Doesn't Know Might Kill You with Dr. Robert Thompson. (Take Charge Books, 2008).

The Secret of Health: Breast Wisdom with Dr. Ben Johnson. (Morgan James Publishing 2007).

User's Guide to Thyroid Disorders. (Basic Health Publications, 2006).

User's Guide to Natural Hormone Replacement. (Basic Health Publications, 2006).

Arthritis and Joint Health. (Woodland Publishing, 2005).

www.ingramcontent.com/pod-product-compliance
Lightning Source LLC
Chambersburg PA
CBHW050545280326
41933CB00011B/1727